ALL NATURAL
FLEA & TICK
PREVENTION PLAN

THE BEST FOOD-BASED PEST PROTECTION FOR DOGS & CATS

JEAN BRANNON

LICENSED ACUPUNCTURIST

CONTENTS

THE PEST PROBLEM

Introduction — 4

Fleas And Ticks Are Like Superhero Pests — 7

Amazing Flea Facts — 9

Troublesome Tick Trivia — 12

The Discouraging Quest For A Truly Effective Natural Pest Protocol — 15

The "Good Ol' Days" Of Flea Baths And Bombs — 17

Years Of Trying – And Failing – To Find A Simpler, Safer Solution — 19

Western Medicine's "Miracle Flea And Tick Pills" — 21

THE HELPFUL TOOLS

Many Holistic Flea And Tick Remedies Mildly Work Sometimes – THIS Natural Protocol Works Dependably Well — 23

What Is "Earthing" – And How Does It Help? — 25

What Is "Structured Water" – And How Does It Help? — 27

We Are All What We Eat — 29

Pests Seek The Weak — 30

Diatomaceous Earth Dices And Dries Pests Soon After Contact — 32

How This Plan Helped Our Dog Beyond Just Flea And Tick Relief — 34

A Dependably Good Flea And Tick Plan — 37

The Truth About Garlic — 38

One Old Study's Misleading Findings Still Harm Garlic's Reputation — 40

Garlic's Many Benefits — 42

To Be An Effective Flea And Tick Preventative, Garlic Must Smell — 44

THE PREVENTION PLAN

Directions And Dosages	47
Additional Thoughts	52
A Species-Appropriate Food Plan	55
Ingredients To Seek – And Ones To Avoid	59
See Your Veterinarian If You're Unsure About Anything	62
About The Author	63

INTRODUCTION

OVER 40 YEARS OF TRIAL AND ERROR LED TO THIS SAFE, SIMPLE, ALL NATURAL FLEA AND TICK SOLUTION . . . THAT REALLY WORKS!

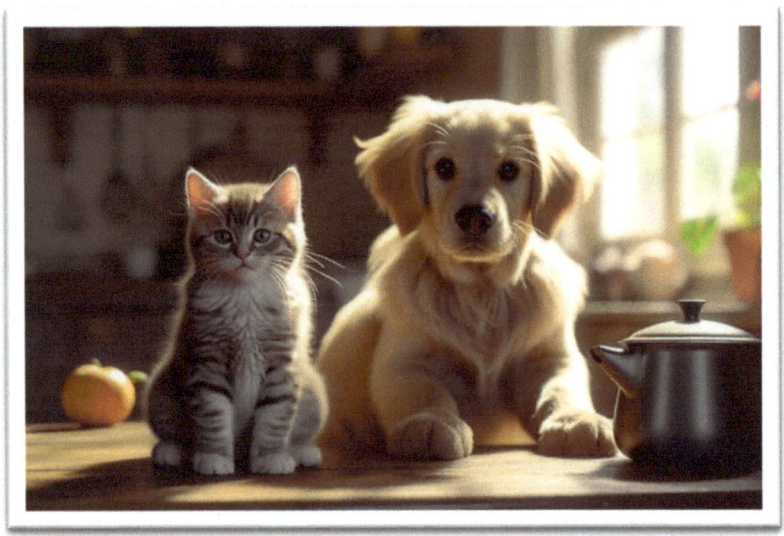

"An ounce of prevention is worth a pound of cure," Benjamin Franklin once famously said. This philosophy echoes Taoist thinking and, in fact, all ancient teachings. From illness to exercising to intervening when a naughty pup ransacks the trash, it's generally wise advice in all matters of life. But perhaps it's never more important than when planning a flea and tick strategy.

If you have pets, I'm sure you understand why prevention is so preferable to cure. Because when you have dogs and cats, you've almost certainly had to try and think ahead sometimes to keep them from eating chocolate or scratching your favorite chairs. And when you have fur kids, you've also most assuredly encountered fleas and ticks – those nasty critters we all love to hate.

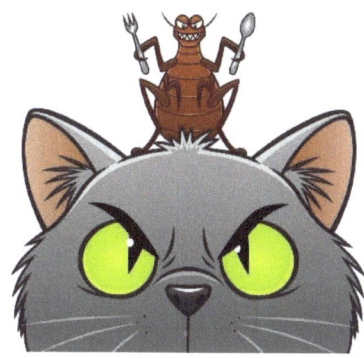

And if you're like me, you've probably failed at some point to prevent fleas and ticks and been forced to find a pound of cure to get rid of them. Perhaps also like me, you've investigated natural potential cures as well as not-so-natural ones. But no matter what I've tried over the years, most flea and tick elimination protocols I've used have serious drawbacks.

The latest chemical control options are decidedly effective at eradicating fleas and ticks. Yet not only are they expensive and need to be continually administered; chemical controls are pesticides, and pesticides are toxic. This kind of toxicity can lead to serious health issues for both pets and people, so I think due diligence is important for anyone looking to use chemical flea and tick control. Please discuss these options with your veterinarian, and also be sure to do your own research, so you can be certain you're well informed about all available options and the choices you make moving forward.

There are also countless natural flea and tick control strategies. I've tried literally every holistic approach I've heard about or that's been recommended to me over the last 40-plus years. In my experience, these remedies often have some merit and yet fall short of being able to eliminate fleas and ticks *dependably*. Natural pest control options are often criticized for being weaker and less effective than chemical methods and, generally speaking, I can't disagree.

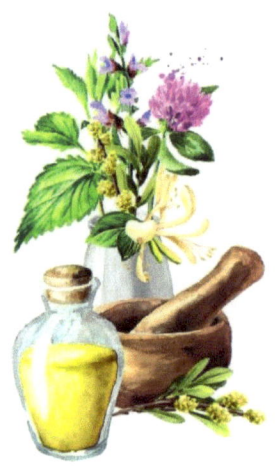

Yet natural approaches *do* work well if you adopt a comprehensive plan and stick to it. In my experience, it took years of trial and error to hit on a combination of just a few holistic remedies that would work together in one simple plan to control fleas and ticks – dependably and naturally!

FLEAS AND TICKS ARE LIKE SUPERHERO PESTS

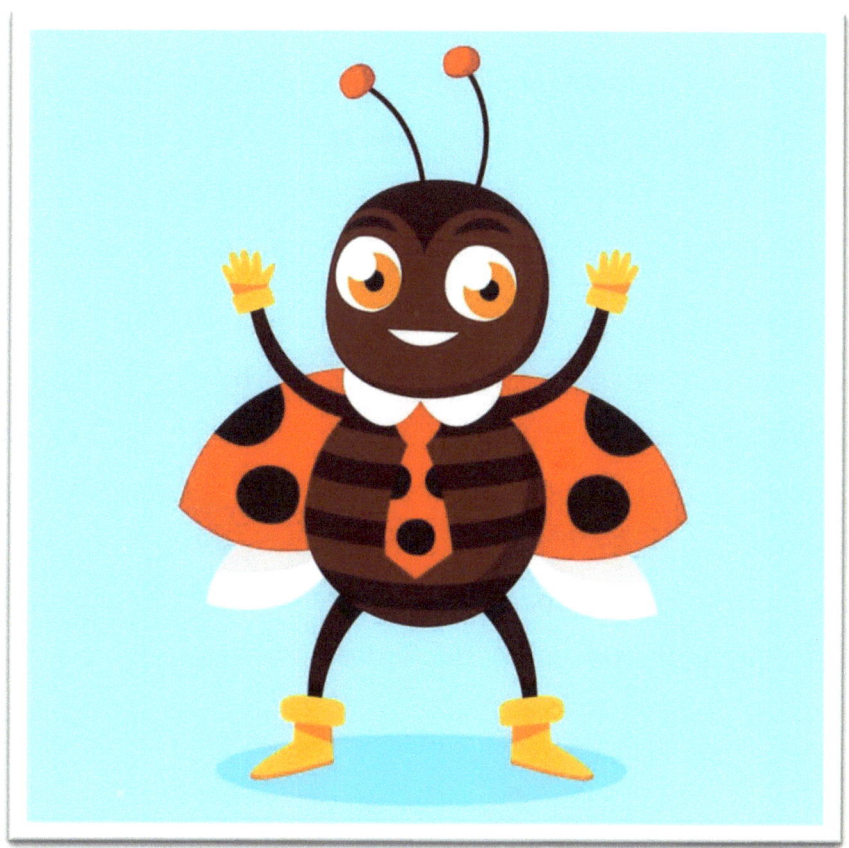

Admittedly, it took me decades to discover a dependably effective natural pest protocol. This delayed discovery is partly due to me feeling bewildered any time I investigated the topic. And that's because the available research on natural flea and tick remedies and repellants is filled with contradictory information. Garlic, brewer's yeast, and apple cider vinegar are three examples of food-based remedies that read either like miraculous cure-alls or dangerous substances to be avoided at all cost depending on what you choose to read about them. Veterinarians don't even agree when it comes to natural flea and tick solutions or their chemical alternatives. And though I've asked all the veterinarians I've trusted over the years about pest-control options, I was still slow to develop this completely natural protocol. Not only did it take me years to sift through books, articles, and journals – but I needed time to keep experimenting with food-based therapies on my own dogs and cats to see what truly helped them the most.

Another reason it took so long to find a **reliably effective** natural preventative is because fleas and ticks are, by their very natures, crafty creatures. They know more than a thing or two about survival. And they've evolved over millions of years into hardy parasites that make the most of every opportunity to exploit our pets (and us). Their sheer adaptability means any approach to controlling them needs to be equally versatile in order to be effective.

AMAZING FLEA FACTS

Consider, for example, that fleas have reportedly been around for about 100 million years. They're wingless insects that have developed over time into more than 2,500 known species. And in most of these flea species, the females are not only bigger than males, but they can eat 15 times their weight in blood every day.

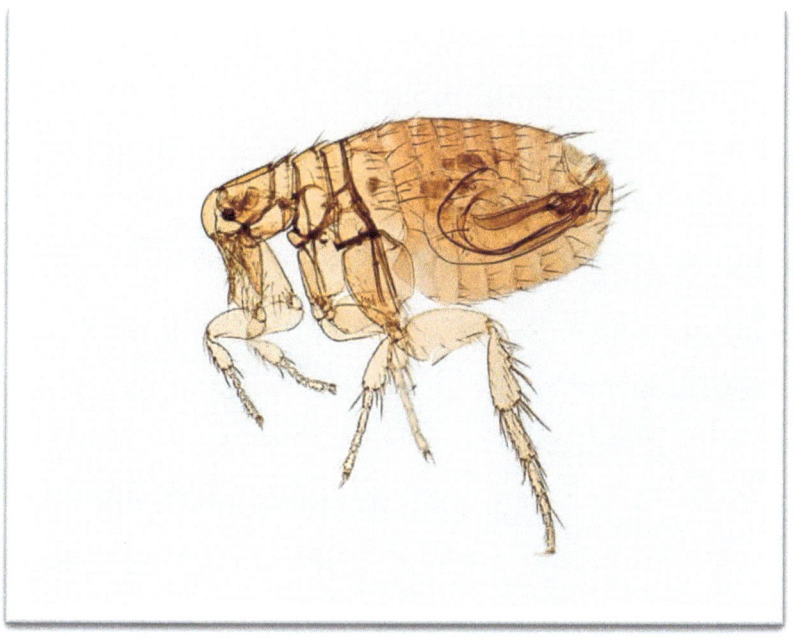

(Illustration by CDC on Unsplash.)

Since each female can live up to three months on a single "blood meal" and can lay up to 2,000 eggs in that time, it's easy to see how flea populations can feast off your pets and explode quickly inside your home if you don't have an effective control plan in place.

Every life stage of the flea shows how it's built to survive. Think about the females laying all those eggs in their 30- to 90-day lifetimes – up to 50 eggs per day. Eggs that are deposited directly onto a living host's body (such as your dog or cat). But these eggs also easily fall off and get spread around into couches and carpets. It then takes between two days and two weeks (depending on factors like temperature and humidity) for eggs to hatch into blind larvae; these larvae then feed off of adult flea waste (commonly referred to as the "flea dirt" found on your pet) before forming a sticky cocoon. This tough, protective shell sticks to fibers, making it not only difficult to vacuum up from carpeting and upholstery – but resistant to chemical flea killers as well.

Inside this cocoon, larvae transform into pupae over the course of about 21 days. Yet pupae won't emerge as adult fleas until a potential host makes itself known. That means rising levels of carbon dioxide, vibration, and heat – all signs exhibited by a living host – must be sensed or else the pupae will remain in the cocoon until conditions are right. And that can be years! (That's why vacuuming sometimes leads to more adult flea sightings, since it can produce enough vibration and heat to signal the pupae that a viable host – and thus a meal – is waiting.) Which can then send masses of new adults streaming out of their cocoons!

Once you begin to realize this vast scope and complexity of a flea's life cycle, it starts to sink in how these unwanted pests can quickly wreak havoc on your household – until you find a way to get rid of them. Which is, admittedly, a daunting task.

By the time you start seeing adult fleas, you need to accept you're only observing maybe five percent of the problem. Adults are evidence, though, of the legions of eggs and emerging pupae that undoubtedly are lurking deep in your rugs and recliners. And it's this hardy and hard to break life cycle that makes combatting an active flea infestation so problematic. Fighting a full-on infestation demands patience and persistence – and it's a dramatic example of how preventing an issue in the first place is always easier (and preferable) to cleaning up a mess that's already been made.

Add to their impressive reproductive capabilities the fact that fleas truly defy physics with their extraordinary physical abilities, and there's simply no denying what formidable foes they are. Able to leap up to 100 times their bodies' own 1/8" length, fleas can also jump around 30,000 times in a row and lift things 150 times heavier than they are. If humans had this level of strength, we'd be able to leap over the Eiffel Tower, using a force 50 times greater than the power needed to launch rockets into space!

TROUBLESOME TICK TRIVIA

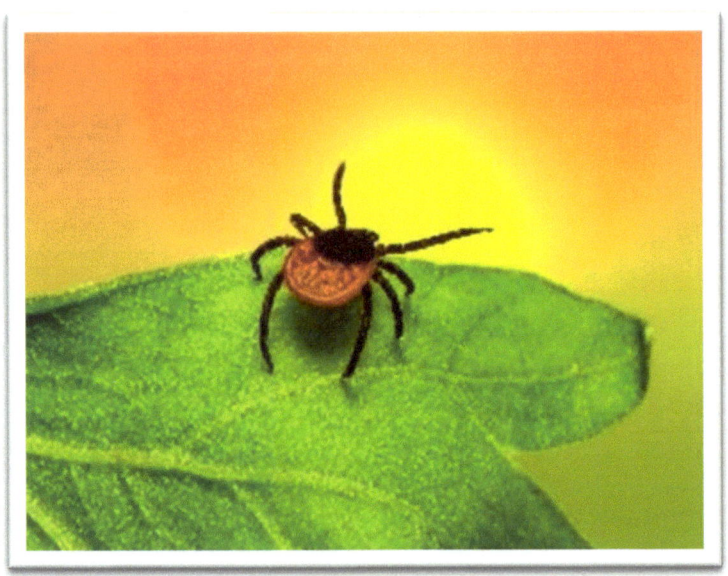

(Photo by Erik Karits on Unsplash.)

As you're likely aware, fleas and ticks have many contrasting characteristics. One difference is that fleas pose more of an indoor issue, whereas ticks by and large are an outdoor problem, since ticks don't set up indoor colonies. Ticks are loners; they tend to wait in tall grasses or hanging foliage to hitch a ride on a hospitable host.

In all, there are about 850 known tick species dating back at least 100 million years. They're classified as *arachnids*, which means they have eight legs and resemble spiders and scorpions more than insects. But somewhat amusingly, ticks are daredevils.

They don't see well and they can't fly, but they do sense their prey long before it arrives because they're quite sensitive to odor, heat, and vibration. When a host is near, ticks will crawl high up and clasp leaves or brush with their back legs. Then they dangle, trying to grab their intended prey with their front legs. Ticks will even leap in a free-fall dive and hope to land on a passing potential host.

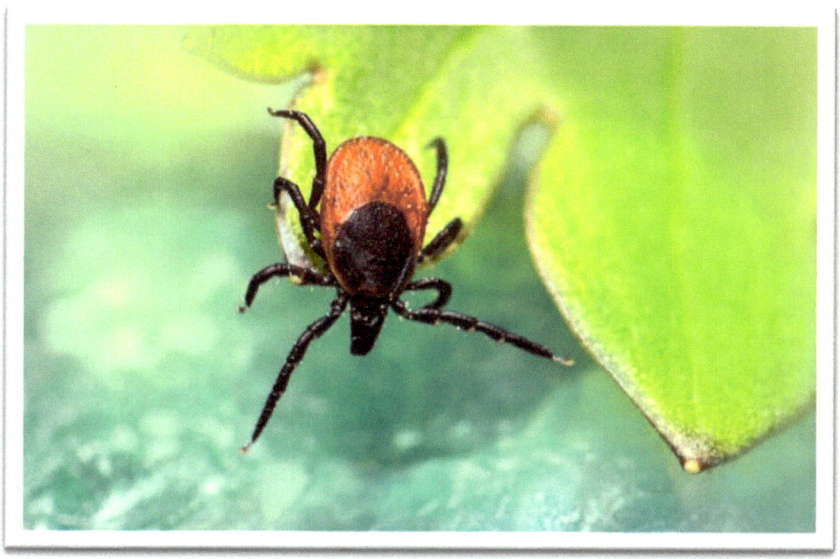

(Photo by Erik Karits on Unsplash.)

Compared to fleas, ticks live a long time and can go very long periods without eating. One African tick species reportedly lived in a lab without any food for eight years! This hardiness is one reason ticks can be challenging to control.

Female ticks become much bigger than males after a meal. Both males and females will often die after mating, but not before the female first lays up to 18,000 eggs.

Known to carry and transmit a host of infections like Lyme disease and Rocky Mountain spotted fever, ticks are slow and methodical feeders once they find a host. Sometimes a tick spends up to two hours preparing a spot where it's chosen to attach. The tick will first bury its head beneath the skin. Then it inserts its feeding tube, using it to spit out blood-thinning and skin-numbing saliva before feasting for up to three days.

A tick's slowness is helpful in that even an infected tick may take eight hours or longer to transmit disease. So if you find an attached tick after an outdoor excursion, it's likely you'll be able to remove it without contracting an illness. That's why carefully checking yourself and your pets for ticks after trips outside is important.

THE DISCOURAGING QUEST FOR A TRULY EFFECTIVE NATURAL PEST PROTOCOL

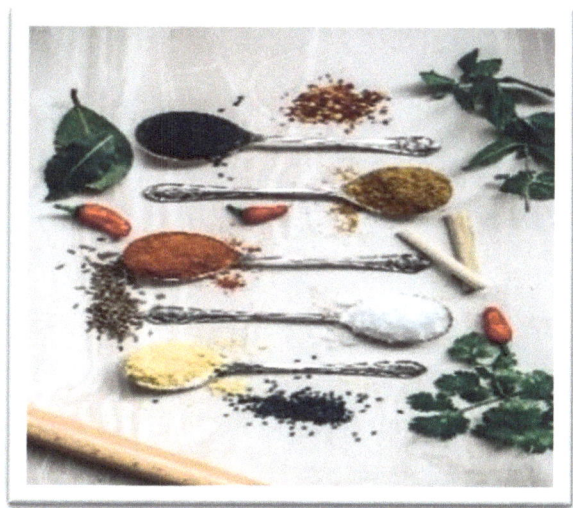

Personally, as an acupuncturist, I prefer natural ways of handling everything, as I do my best to live holistically and according to nature's principles. Yet I spent years trying any and all holistic flea and tick prevention remedies and strategies I read or heard about – to no avail. Honestly, after a while I felt like Goldilocks ... this one's too harsh, this one's too weak, and this one's just a "why bother at all".

And I got really discouraged. I truly didn't like resorting to chemical flea control methods, although at one point my family and I moved with our dog to Florida. And southwest Florida never gets consistently cold enough for long enough to break the flea cycle. Unfortunately, our pup became so miserable with constant itching and scabs and hair loss that we resorted to chemicals at our new place. The effect was immediate; within hours, our dog had completely stopped scratching and licking and biting herself. We all slept better after that, and it was without a doubt an effective approach to flea control. But a *safe* one?

I felt uneasy using these undeniably powerful – and powerfully toxic – substances. Just reading the directions and accompanying warnings gave me the shivers. And yet I'd tried so many natural remedies for so many years – and nothing ever seemed to work anywhere nearly as well as the chemicals so obviously did. I thought back to the days I'd experienced before more recent breakthroughs in chemical flea prevention. Back then, it seemed like nothing at all would ever work to solve flea infestations, as even chemical preventatives didn't seem any more effective than their natural alternatives.

THE "GOOD OL' DAYS" OF FLEA BATHS AND BOMBS

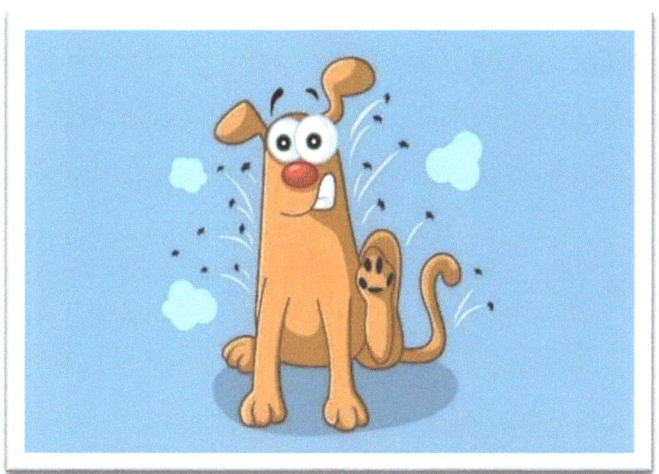

When I think back to 1977 – the year my family got its first puppy – we for sure had no idea how persnickety (and persistent!) fleas actually were. Where we lived in rural West Virginia, western veterinary medicine recommended a flea collar and flea dip approach. (Do you remember those chalky white "Hartz two-in-one collars"? The ones that in our experience truly turned out to be in the "why bother" camp?)

Well, we couldn't find any other options, so we followed this protocol religiously. Yet our pooch still struggled with intense itching and hot spots and obsessive licking; clearly, she stayed in distress throughout the summer months despite our best efforts. I remember being fascinated by how fleas could hop onto us from where they'd somehow created a mostly invisible stronghold – from carpets to the couch.

Yet when we bathed our Maltese terrier (a weekly affair), I couldn't believe how quickly and easily fleas drowned! We always applied the flea dip afterward and put that darned Hartz collar back on and continued the daily flea-combing and vacuuming rituals, but these efforts never actually solved the problem. An hour after bathtime, Mitzi would be scratching like crazy. And it was awful to see how little relief she got from this "flea hell" despite all we were doing to help her.

YEARS OF TRYING – AND FAILING – TO FIND A SIMPLER, SAFER SOLUTION

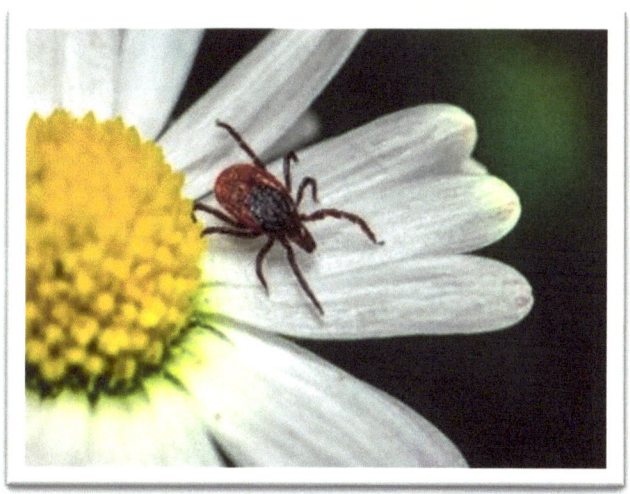

(Photo by Erik Karits on Unsplash.)

I was just a kid at the time, but I felt in my heart there MUST be a better way to deal with fleas and ticks that actually *worked*. Over the coming years, we did find and try different flea collars and flea dip brands, but nothing had a lasting effect. I'd always read every label obsessively to make sure my sister and I (as the volunteer pup bathers) were doing everything correctly. And while I was sure we were following all the instructions, I still had that despairing feeling about all the label warnings; they spelled out so many potential health risks (for both pooches AND people) from using these admittedly toxic chemicals.

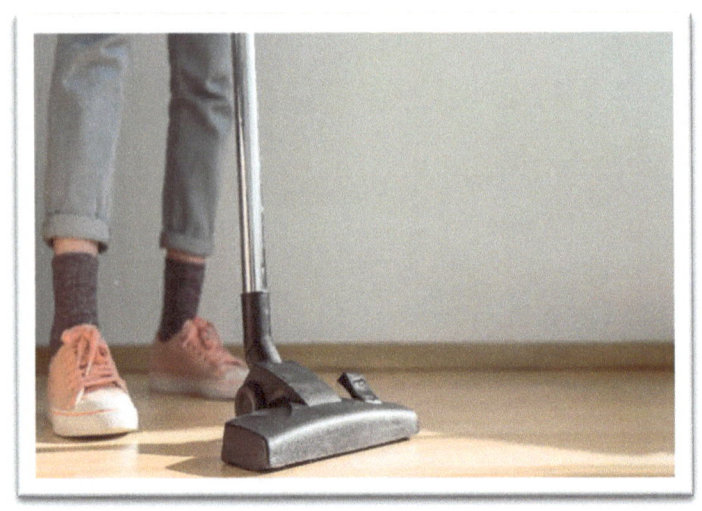

(Image by Freepik.)

Regardless, we kept up the spring and summer bathing and dipping and occasional flea bombing (plus daily combing and vacuuming), since we really didn't know what else to do. I couldn't believe how many fleas we sucked up in the vacuum either! We tore into a full vacuum bag one time just out of curiosity – and then we ran screaming when TONS of fleas hopped to freedom all over and around us!

Finally, a neighbor gave us a tip to put moth balls into the vacuum bag to kill captured fleas. This trick seemed to work well, so we endured the nasty sweeper smell all summer long. But we'd only breathe a real sigh of relief after fall's first killing frost, because that icy temperature truly seemed to break the flea cycle – and return our household peace for at least winter's duration.

WESTERN MEDICINE'S "MIRACLE FLEA AND TICK PILLS"

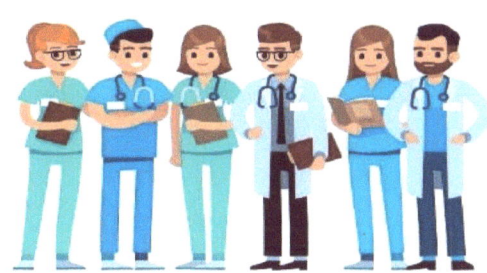

A few years later, many of our relatives started using western veterinary medicine's oral flea and tick drugs, and I remember how elated everyone felt to stop obsessive flea combing and all the topical treatments and daily vacuuming. Certainly, this approach is effective, and many people these days still opt to use these types of treatments to manage all sorts of pet pests. (For sure, I used this method myself while living in Florida, as I've already shared.)

Yet as I embraced an increasingly holistic approach to life, I kept researching natural flea and tick prevention options. I really wanted to find something natural that could equal the latest evolution in chemical solutions. As part of my acupuncture schooling, I learned a lot about herbs as well as other supplements. Since childhood, I'd never stopped experimenting with every alternative flea and tick remedy that came into my awareness. But once I became a licensed acupuncturist – and as a pet parent to three rescue dogs and three rescue cats – I began a deep dive into all I'd been learning to see if I could find the simplest, most effective, and most affordable way to eliminate flea and tick worries … naturally!

MANY HOLISTIC FLEA AND TICK REMEDIES MILDLY WORK SOMETIMES – THIS NATURAL PROTOCOL WORKS DEPENDABLY WELL

One truth I've found throughout my holistic training and clinical practice is this – very, *very* few things work 100 percent of the time for everybody and everything in every situation. In my opinion, that means the rare remedies and methods that DO work dependably well are important to use.

An example of something that helps nearly every imbalance leading to lack of vitality and illness is the process of *earthing*, or connecting to the earth by placing one's bare feet on the ground (or by gardening without gloves). In harsh weather or for folks confined to hospital beds or for cats kept inside all the time, grounding mats and other earthing tools to use indoors may be found at www.earthing.com.

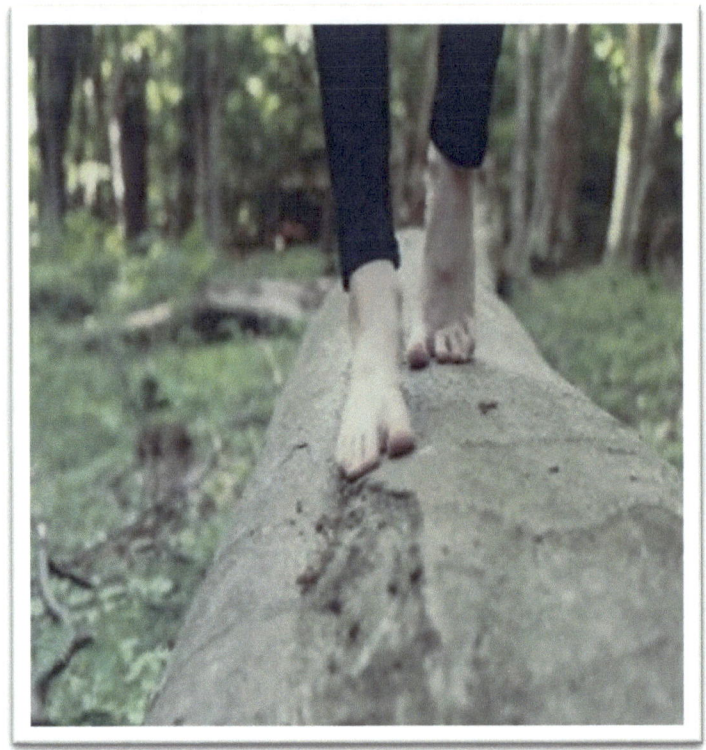

Please understand I'm not being paid by anyone at this site to spread awareness about earthing or to endorse their products. But I am one of their customers, and I believe this company's documentary is one of the very best introductions and explorations of earthing I've ever seen. I'm providing a link for you to check it out for yourself here: www.earthingmovie.com.

WHAT IS "EARTHING" – AND HOW DOES IT HELP?

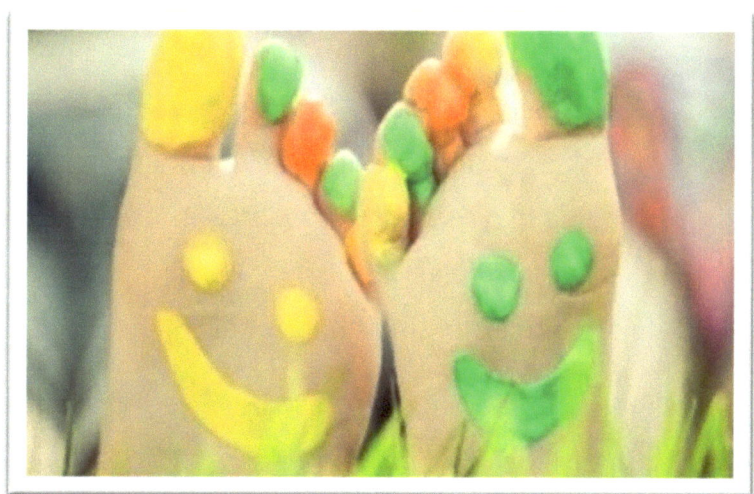

I do hope you'll watch the documentary, but in short, I'd like to describe what earthing is and why it's so important to overall health for people and pets alike. A very simple way of explaining earthing is to equate it with how electricity works.

For example, a properly grounded outlet supplies safe and instantaneous power when you plug a cord into it. Similarly, our bare feet – if nothing blocks them from contacting the earth's surface directly – will connect to the earth's electromagnetic current as soon as we place our bare skin to the ground. And while we are thus "plugged in", our bodies (which are essentially electromagnetically powered) gain not only beneficial electrical energies the earth freely gives; our systems also can discharge accumulated stress and its accompanying inflammation right out through our feet. All we need to do is simply allow the earth to absorb (and then transform into positive energies) what we release.

So as you can see from this description, earthing is a stunningly simple concept. Yet it's so easy to do that people often dismiss just how positively earthing can affect health and well-being. For sure, sick or injured animals instinctively know to curl up on the ground, which helps to direct inflammation out of their bodies. See how those daily dog walks are more than simply bathroom breaks? They're doggy earthing opportunities!

In past times, people widely knew how healing it was to go barefoot. Before the practice of wearing shoes became so widespread, there was much less chronic disease in the world. If you research earthing's benefits, you'll discover that no scientific studies have ever disproven its ability to help any bodily imbalance, which is why I've long recommended it to my acupuncture patients.

WHAT IS "STRUCTURED WATER" – AND HOW DOES IT HELP?

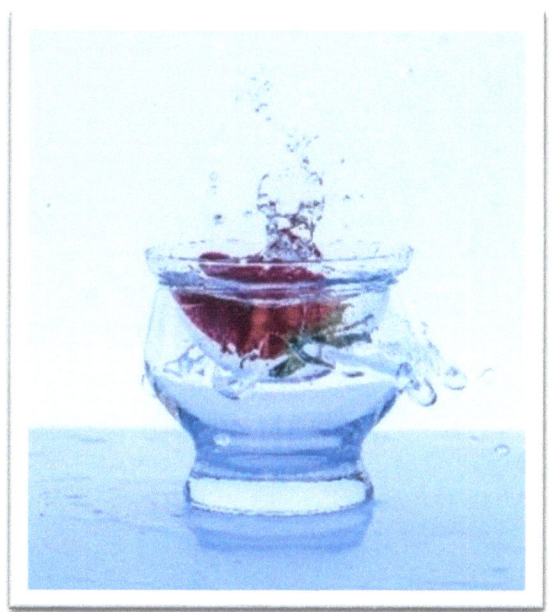

In addition to earthing, another tool I've found that works for nearly everyone (people as well as pets) is proper daily hydration. The very best way to hydrate is to drink enough water, which for humans equates to drinking half one's body weight in ounces every day. (For example, a 100-pound person would need to drink 50 ounces of water daily in order to be hydrated enough to carry out basic metabolic functions in an efficient manner.)

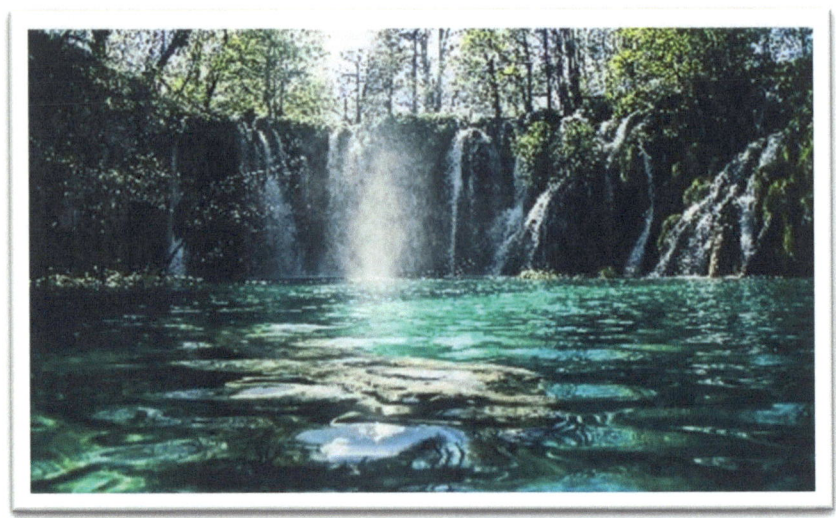

In nature, water running in rivers and waterfalls becomes electrically charged from the energy such movement infuses into it; this type of water is called *structured water*, and it's been shown to be so much more hydrating and cell supporting than tap water. Around the world, many bodies of water deemed to be sacred and to carry healing energies are actually structured water sites (such as Lourdes in France). And so for those who use city tap water instead of natural spring water, I believe choosing a water filtration system that structures as well as purifies and alkalizes the water can be highly beneficial for humans as well as pets. (Please do your own diligent research to learn more.)

WE ARE ALL WHAT WE EAT

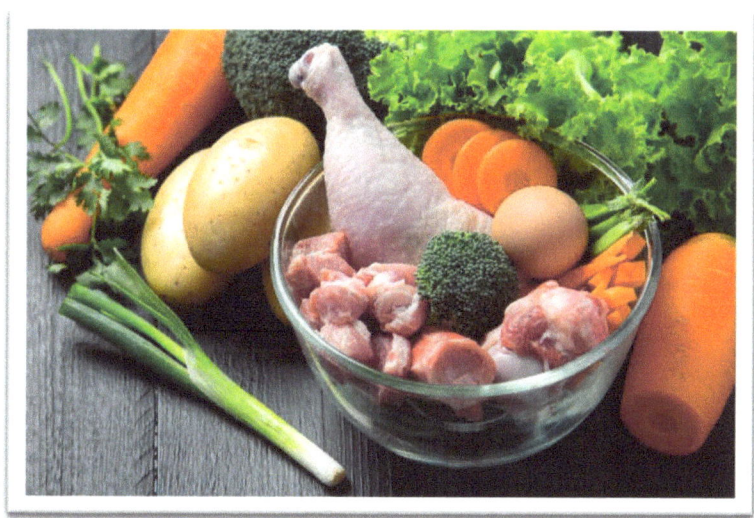

As I've described, I believe part of an effective natural flea and tick protocol involves letting pets have access to the earth and plenty of fresh structured water. Yet another key element is feeding a species-appropriate diet, one without processed fillers and artificial ingredients. (I've found that a non-GMO, grain-free, raw-coated kibble along with organ-meat-plus-tripe wet foods are a very helpful feeding foundation for most dogs and cats, for instance.) I also feed my pups raw meaty bones to keep their teeth clean and to provide needed enzymes for their bodies – just like they'd eat in the wild. Yet what supplements can be added to this wellness plan to address fleas and ticks specifically?

PESTS SEEK THE WEAK

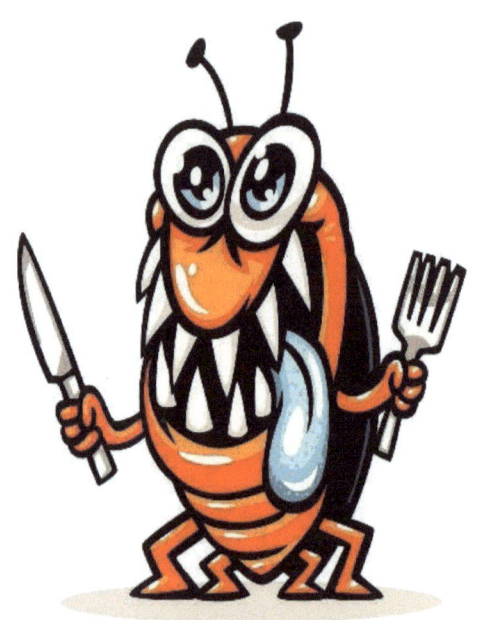

It's really important to understand that fleas and ticks are parasites, and as such, they "feed" off of their hosts (meaning our pets). A key point most holistically minded veterinarians will make is that a pet with a healthy immune system who's active and eats a good "species-appropriate" diet is much less susceptible to fleas and ticks in the first place. But even healthy dogs and cats are likely to pick up fleas and ticks if they spend any time at all outdoors.

In my years of experimenting with flea and tick supplements looking for a "magic bullet", I've found lots of supplements to be at least partially helpful (if not 100% effective for all pets).

Brewer's yeast and garlic powder added to a pet's food every day is enough to repel fleas and ticks dependably in some animals (especially cats) as a solo treatment – but it's not going to work just by itself in many animals.

DIATOMACEOUS EARTH DICES AND DRIES PESTS SOON AFTER CONTACT

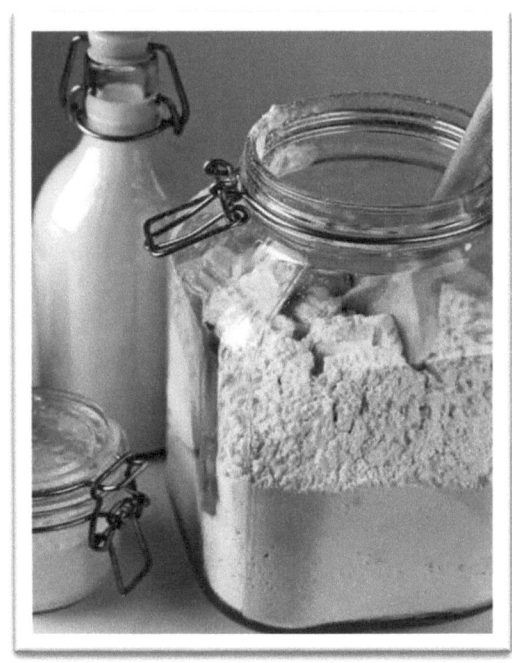

(Photo by Kristiana Pinne on Unsplash.)

Diatomaceous earth is another powerful remedy for killing parasites – including fleas. It's the only known treatment that works as a physical agent to break down adult flea bodies. If you use diatomaceous earth topically, you can watch it start to dry up fleas or ticks on contact. It's made of tiny crushed shells that are harmless to people or pets when eaten, yet most parasites cannot survive diatomaceous earth's cutting nature and dehydrate soon after contact.

If you read up on diatomaceous earth, you'll find many skeptics claim it's not effective against all pet parasites. What I've found is it isn't powerful enough used by itself against fleas, because on its own, it can't break the flea's life cycle. Yet it's a crucial part of this protocol I'm sharing with you, because its mechanical ability to dry up insects is unique.

If diatomaceous earth is combined with just a few additional food-based supplements and an overall healthy nutrition plan, it becomes a key component of an effective natural flea and tick prevention strategy; this food-based approach not only helps control fleas and ticks – it promotes overall vitality as well.

Currently, in our own household, we have a "United Nations" of mixed dog breeds along with a full-blooded Great Pyrenees rescue. Our smallest mixed terrier/shepherd pup weighs 40 pounds, and our Great Pyrenees is quite a big boy at more than 150 pounds. We also have a basset hound mix, a golden retriever mix, and another shepherd mix. All of these dogs differ wildly in terms of temperament, skin sensitivity, and fur texture.

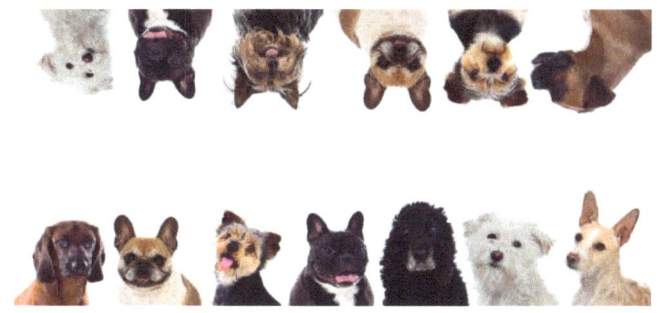

HOW THIS PLAN HELPED OUR DOG BEYOND JUST FLEA AND TICK RELIEF

Our "delicate lotus blossom", though, had for years been our golden retriever mix Connell. We learned that, as a puppy, he'd been given a mange vaccine that somehow made his immune system go haywire. And so I spent over three years (and several thousand dollars) seeking nutrition therapy and homeopathic veterinary assistance, yet nothing really helped his painful skin that was covered in bald spots and weeping sores.

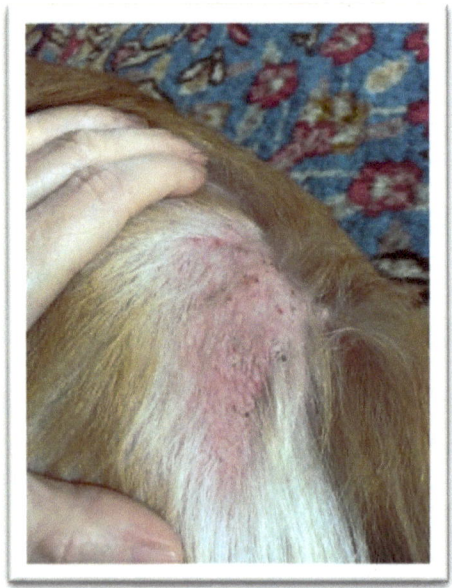

(2017 photo showing scabs in one of Connell's bald spots.)

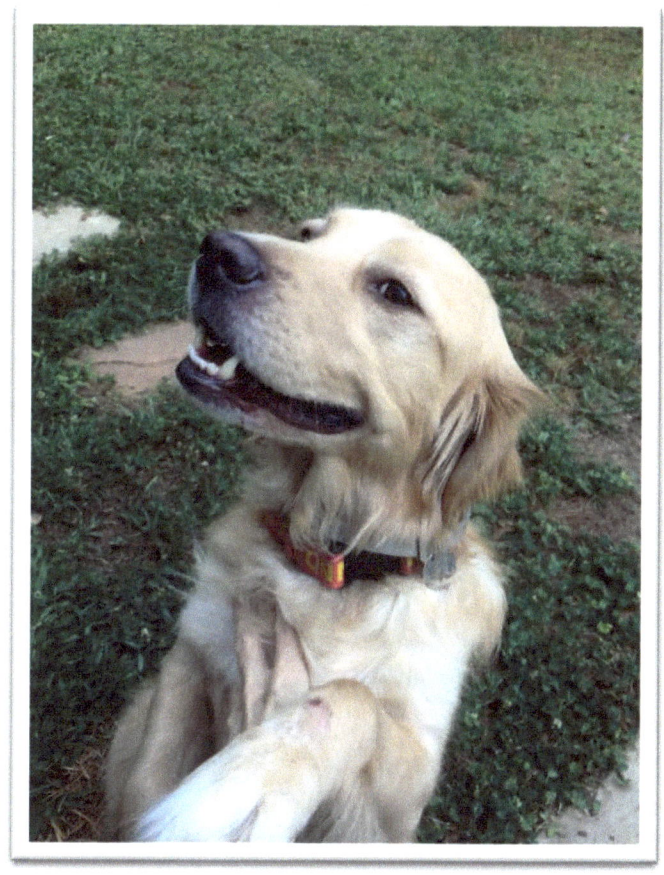

(2017 photo showing a sore on Connell's paw and his sparse coat.)

It wasn't until I hit on the three key supplements needed for natural flea and tick control that Connell's overall health turned a corner. Once I got him on this regimen and a tripe-based, raw meaty bones diet (complete details come later in this book), he fully recovered in about three months' time. For several years now, he's had the most beautiful golden coat – and his feet and legs are tufted with lovely feathery fluff. He's still vibrantly healthy and going strong at over 10 years old!

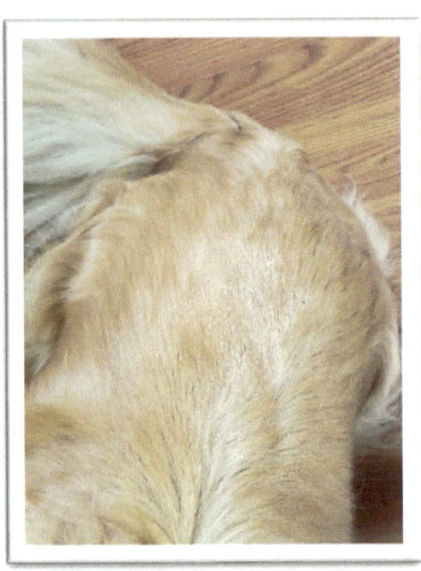

(2024 photo showing Connell's completely healed back with full and shiny coat.)

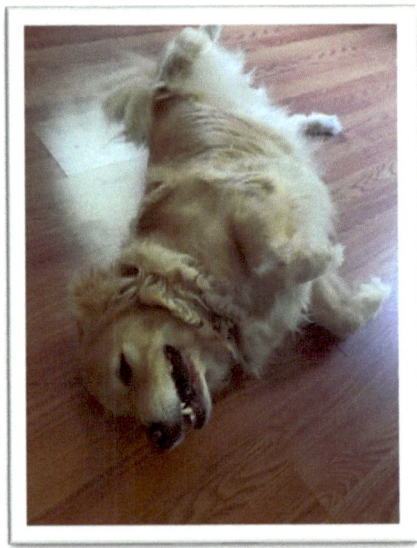

(2024 photo showing Connell with a thick and lustrous coat and no irritated skin.)

A DEPENDABLY GOOD FLEA AND TICK PLAN

This pest protocol's recommended dosages should be adjusted based upon pet weight; any new supplementation regimen or dietary change needs to be adopted slowly over the course of a few weeks. Please understand I'm not sharing this protocol as a substitute for sound veterinary advice, and it is in no way intended to replace quality veterinary care. Please see your veterinarian immediately if you feel your pet needs attention.

Also, please note that I receive no compensation from the companies whose supplements or foods I recommend; I share what I've learned over the years from my own experiences and from patients and friends sharing their experiences. There are many good supplement companies, so please do your own research and make choices based upon what feels best for you and your pets.

THE TRUTH ABOUT GARLIC

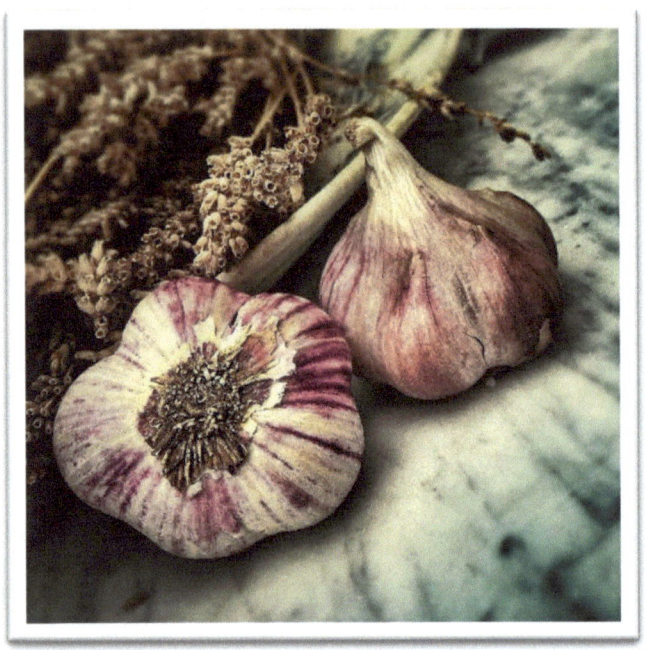

(Photo by Lobo Studio Hamburg on Unsplash.)

I can't think of a single natural substance that's more misunderstood in holistic pet care than garlic. I've studied garlic extensively as an acupuncturist, and I've talked about it with the many veterinarians I've consulted personally in more than 40 years of being a pet parent. If you do careful research, you'll see there's nothing in any of the available literature to indicate that garlic per se is toxic to dogs or cats. Every single book I've consulted that includes sections on herbal pet remedies recommends garlic for pets. Then why, you might ask, is there a lot of misinformation out there (and some of it is even touted by veterinarians) that makes it sound like it's downright dangerous to give garlic to our fur kids? The answer is that most evidence-based research doesn't know what to do with a "food as medicine" approach. As such, accurately quantifying all of the variables inherent in studying whole plant medicines makes this process tricky. Most research studies I've come across base their findings on garlic extracts lacking raw garlic's potent enzymes and nutrients; these studies also often use what I feel are unreasonably high doses.

Adding to this confusion over garlic's safety is its close association with its sulfur-based "cousins" in the lily family that DO cause harm in dogs – namely onions, leeks, shallots, and chives. But garlic is the only family member that *lacks* problematic levels of the sulfur called *thiosulfate*.

In fact, the thiosulfate found in garlic is in barely traceable amounts, and what's present is readily excreted. Nutritionist Dr. Dave Summers claims that testing reveals how onions have about 15 times the ability of garlic to damage a dog's red blood cells. And so if dogs take in a large amount of thiosulfate from eating onions, leeks, shallots, or chives, this consumption may, over time, lead to a type of anemia called *hemolytic anemia* that could prove fatal. Cats are even more adversely affected, being up to six to eight times more sensitive to onions than dogs are.

ONE OLD STUDY'S MISLEADING FINDINGS STILL HARM GARLIC'S REPUTATION

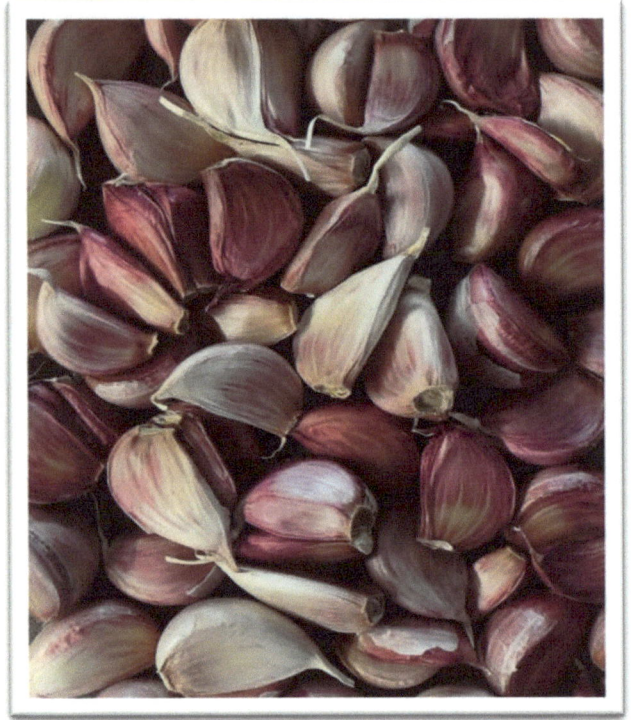

(Photo by Joe Green on Unsplash.)

Perhaps the most infamous garlic safety study in dogs ever conducted that raised an alarm also used alarmingly high dosages. The 2000 study took place in Japan, when K.W. Lee (et al) fed 5 grams of garlic per kilo per day for one week to the dogs in this study. Basically, they found it could be harmful to feed the equivalent of about 60 garlic cloves a day to a 75-pound golden retriever. Well, who would ever even attempt to feed a dog this much garlic? Yet that study has helped fuel the myth that garlic harms dogs, even though the U.S. Federal Department of Agriculture has long approved garlic as a safe pet food ingredient. Fortunately, later research has debunked the misleading 2000 study, such as Dr. Osamu Yamamoto's 2018 study that fed much smaller amounts over a longer period (12 weeks instead of seven days). This study gave only 90 mg per kilo per day, and concluded that this garlic dosage over three months showed no adverse effects at all in dogs.

So what might be considered a "reasonable amount" for pet owners to feed their dogs and cats as a daily flea and tick preventative? Famous homeopathic veterinarian Dr. Richard Pitcairn recommends up to ¼ clove for cats and to use weight as a guide for dogs, with no more than three cloves a day for the largest breeds (100 pounds and over). In her book "The Complete Herbal Book for the Dog", Juliette de Bairacli Levy recommends roughly ½ clove per every 10 to 15 pounds.

GARLIC'S MANY BENEFITS

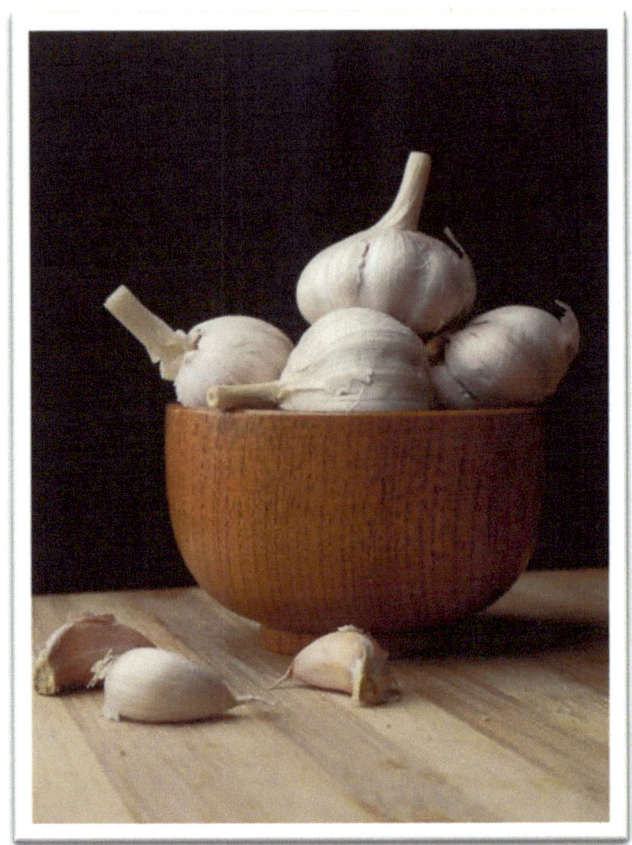

Keep in mind that garlic is *very* different from its onion and leek cousins, and it can help you as well as your fur kids to be more vibrantly healthy. **Overall**, garlic has been recognized as generally safe and beneficial for thousands of years – and not simply as a recipe enhancer. Early Egyptians, Asian doctors, and indigenous cultures around the world have all used garlic for its immune-boosting properties. More recently, modern research supports what ancient wisdom has always known about garlic and touts multiple benefits in people as well as pets. Garlic's nearly magical properties include everything from preventing blood clots, arterial plaque, and tumors to powerful antibiotic, anti-fungal, and anti-parasitic capabilities.

In Chinese medicine's herbology, garlic is classified as a warming and pungent herb. According to Chinese food therapy principles, warmth encourages digestion, while the pungent flavor has a dispersing action that moves energy. Thus, foods and herbs that support digestion and move energy make wonderful additions to a pet's diet not only to aid nutrients in being better absorbed – but to help move parasites (like tapeworms possibly introduced through flea bites) out of a pet's bowel before they can set up housekeeping.

When dogs ingest garlic daily, the sulfur is excreted through the animal's skin even as it collects in natural hair and fur oils; this continual (but not noticeable to a human) presence of a smelly skin and hair barrier forms a key part of an overall natural flea and tick prevention strategy that really works.

TO BE AN EFFECTIVE FLEA AND TICK PREVENTATIVE, GARLIC MUST SMELL

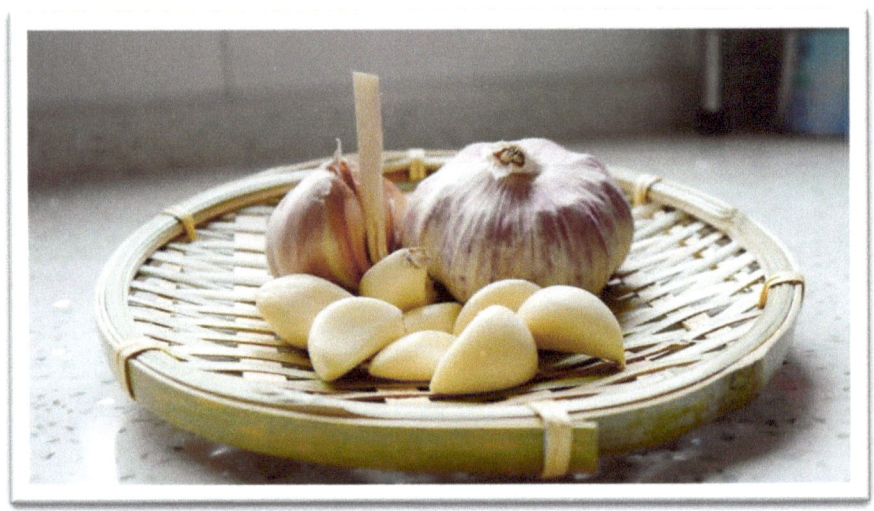

(Photo by Ji Jiali on Unsplash.)

In addition to being rich in amino acids and many nutrients like zinc and vitamin C, garlic owes its nearly miraculous medicinal attributes to its sulfur content. *Allin* is garlic's odor-giving sulfur protein, and *allinase* is its accompanying enzyme. When garlic is crushed or chopped or chewed, the allinase enzyme acts on and combines with the allin protein to produce *allicin*, which is the activated and thus therapeutic form of garlic. It's important to wait at least 10 minutes after mincing garlic to give it to your pets so you can be assured the enzymatic action is complete. (If you're preparing garlic to be cooked in a recipe, you'll still want to wait 10 minutes after chopping it to proceed; that way, you'll be assured you get allicin's benefits because allicin is heat stable once its enzymatic transformation has occurred.)

Even though I believe it's almost always better to use a food or herb in its raw form whenever possible, let me also say that I realize we all sometimes find ourselves short on time. And sometimes the very last thing we feel like doing at the end of a very long day is peeling and chopping raw garlic. (At the time of this writing, I have five large dogs – the smallest is 40 pounds – and so that means when I use raw garlic in our daily protocol, I am chopping a lot of garlic!) I wholeheartedly admit that sometimes I don't take the time to prepare raw garlic, and it's my busy lifestyle that led me to research garlic supplements that could be effective substitutes for those times when prepping garlic just ain't happening.

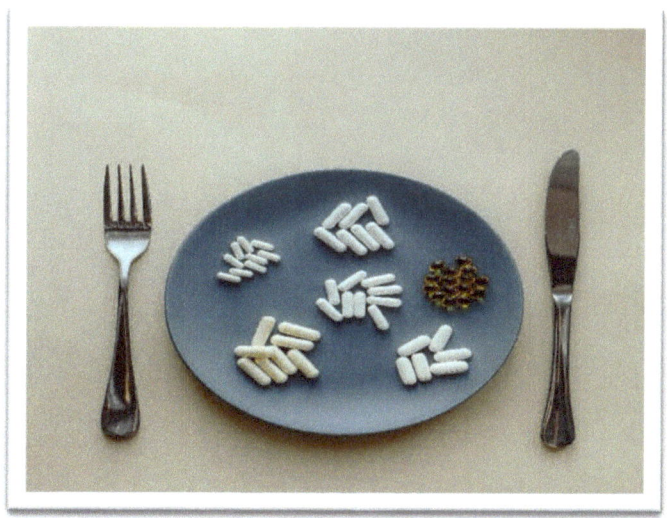

(Photo by Natali Hordiiuk on Unsplash.)

Acupuncturists everywhere who prescribe herbs will likely agree with the philosophy that it's best to find an herbal form an acupuncture patient finds easy to use – because herbs sitting in a cabinet never even get a chance to work. And so that can mean prescribing tea pills or easily dissolved granules instead of the more traditionally revered dried or raw herbs that must be prepared as a tea. Or in the case of this flea and tick protocol, I felt it was important to find and recommend an effective garlic supplement as opposed to raw cloves only.

Basically, my own experimentation over the years correlates with research findings – almost all garlic supplements are ineffective. And all of the odorless ones are completely useless in my experience for this protocol; as soon as the smell is removed, garlic's magical flea- and tick-repelling properties are destroyed.

DIRECTIONS AND DOSAGES

In this section, I've included all the dosages I use for natural foods as well as the supplements I buy from *Amazon*, although you may find quality supplements offered for sale close to where you live instead. I've listed dosages for a 50-70-pound dog; adjust dosages up or down depending on your dog's weight. A 25-pound dog, for example, would require half of the recommended dosage.

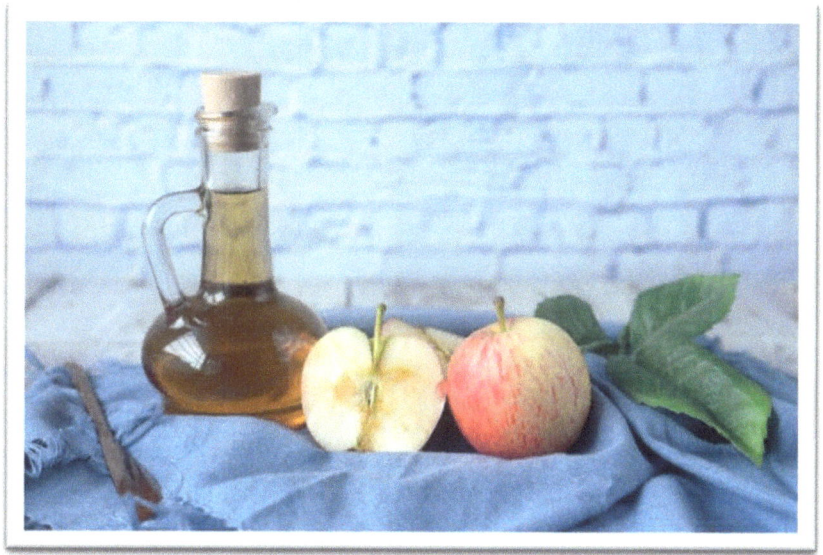

(Photo by Towfiqu Barbhuiya on Unsplash.)

For a 50-70-pound dog: Feed twice a day for the first two months, then reduce to once a day as maintenance. Stir 1 teaspoon of organic, raw, unfiltered apple cider vinegar (I often use *Fairchild's* brand) into the powders listed below along with 1 to 2 tablespoons or more of organic bone broth (I recommend making bone broth the way all our grandmas used to do – from a roasted poultry carcass – but sometimes we don't take the time to make bone broth. So an organic one from your grocery store will work well, too.) Then add the blended powders to some wet pet food before mixing into your dog's regular food.

If using raw garlic, chop 2 cloves if your dog is closer to 50 pounds, and use 3 cloves if your dog is closer to 70 pounds. Personally, I tend to follow the ½ clove per every 10 to 15 pound rule, yet I'm not militant about exact dosages.

If using a supplement, I recommend *Puritan's Pride Garlic Oil 5,000 MG Softgels* (as I mentioned earlier, any garlic used MUST contain pure, smelly garlic oil – deodorized garlic won't work, because it's the odor that keeps adult fleas and ticks from hopping onto your pet):

1. Give one of these odorous softgels hidden in a little canned dog food by hand as a pre-meal treat.

If your pup is one who likes to spit out pills, you can wrap this softgel in a small ball of beef tallow, and it's impossible for it not to be swallowed. You can alternatively pierce the softgel carefully with a knife and squeeze it into wet food. I've found most dogs get used to the taste, and sometimes this way of administering an adequate garlic dosage is easier and more convenient than getting pills into a pup.

2. *Diatomaceous Earth's Organic Food-Grade Diatomaceous Earth Powder*: 1 ½ teaspoons.

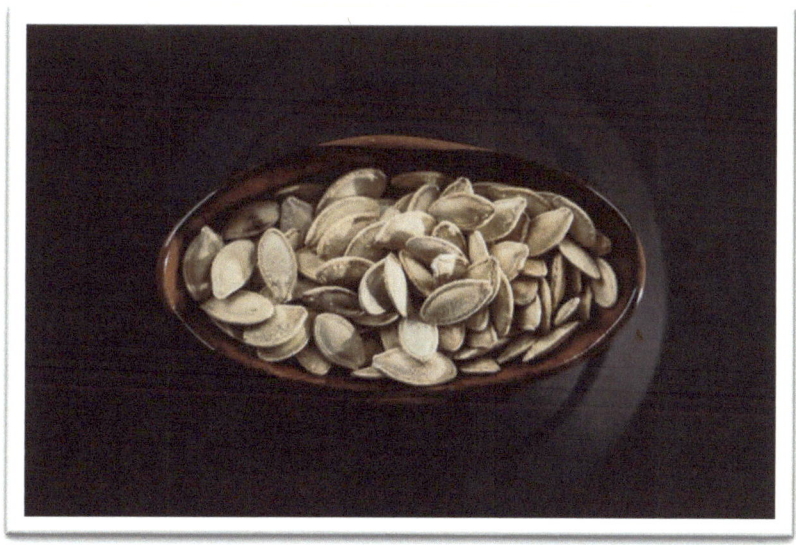

(Photo by Engin Akyurt on Unsplash.)

3. *Horbaach Organic Pumpkin Seed Powder* (this supplement keeps tapeworms from attaching to the intestinal wall, and since you can't have a flea cycle without tapeworms, pumpkin seed powder is crucial to breaking the flea cycle): 1 ½ teaspoons added to diatomaceous earth in a bowl.

4. *Nature's Farmacy 100% Brewer's Yeast And Garlic Powder* (be sure to use a brand with no fillers added): 1 ½ teaspoons.

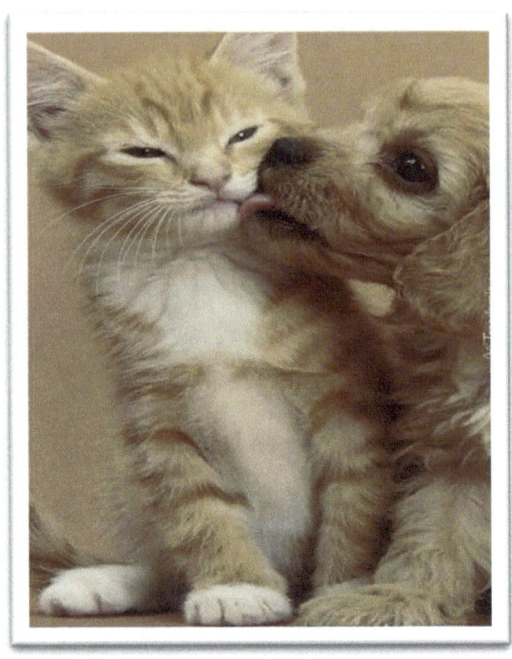

For cats: Eliminate the garlic oil softgel**s** used in the dog protocol. Feed the powders listed below mixed into wet food twice daily with ¼ teaspoon raw apple cider vinegar and topped with *Solid Gold Bone Broth Meal Topper* (available at www.Chewy.com) for the first two months; then reduce to once a day as maintenance. Recommended powder dosages for an average 8- to 12-pound cat are listed. Many cats will eat these recommended powders readily, yet others won't. Try mixing the powders into water-packed, wild-caught sardines if your cat is finicky. In my experience, there's something highly palatable to felines about *Solid Gold's Bone Broth Meal Topper* (and many online reviewers claim that their cats truly find it to be delicious, too). Between sardines and *Solid Gold's* broth, it shouldn't be difficult to get your cats to consume these powders.

1. Food-grade diatomaceous earth powder: ½ teaspoon.

2. Organic pumpkin seed powder: ½ teaspoon.

3. *Strawfield Pets' L-Lysine Immune Support Powder*: 1 scoop. (Be sure to choose a brand with no fillers or sugar added – www.Chewy.com is where we buy ours.)

4. Brewer's yeast and garlic powder: ½ teaspoon. My aunt fed stray cats for many years with a little "side plate" of brewer's yeast and garlic powder, and she said she never found any fleas on any of these kitties. Many cats love the way this powder tastes and will simply eat it right from a plate or sprinkled over kibble; if not, it's usually readily eaten if mixed into wet food.

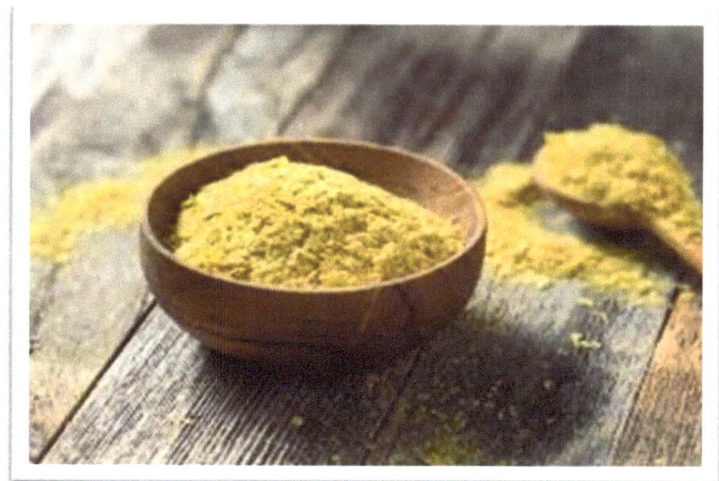

ADDITIONAL THOUGHTS

Natural remedies often take time to work; please be patient, and allow your pets' bodies and immune systems to adjust slowly to a new food and supplement regimen. In my experience in dealing naturally with fleas and ticks, it's easiest to begin the recommended protocol in winter (while temperatures remain at least mostly below freezing – and before warmer temperatures explode the outdoor flea and tick populations).

If you can transform your pets' bodies into "inhospitable hosts" before spring, then you likely won't see a flea at all in your home anymore. And so starting any later than March doesn't mean this approach won't work; it simply means you'll need to keep a closer eye out for up to six to eight weeks to give the supplements enough time to kick in. During this "adjustment period", please know that you could very well have an active flea infestation in your home if you've never successfully kept fleas under control via diligent cleaning methods and natural remedies or by conventional chemical protocols.

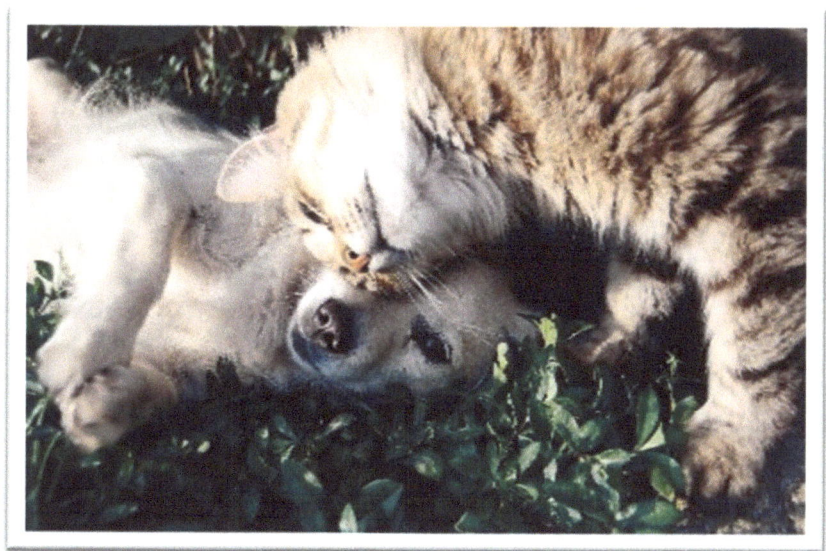

Please make sure you vacuum daily and do a thorough flea combing after any outside visits your fur kids make. It's important to remember, as I've detailed earlier in these pages, that while vacuuming removes fleas, it doesn't kill them. (To prevent fleas from crawling out of the bag once you've finished vacuuming, you can put ¼ cup diatomaceous earth and ¼ cup Neem powder into your vacuum cleaner bag. These powders are a healthier alternative to using moth balls in your vacuum like I did as a kid, and in my experience, these powders are just as effective).

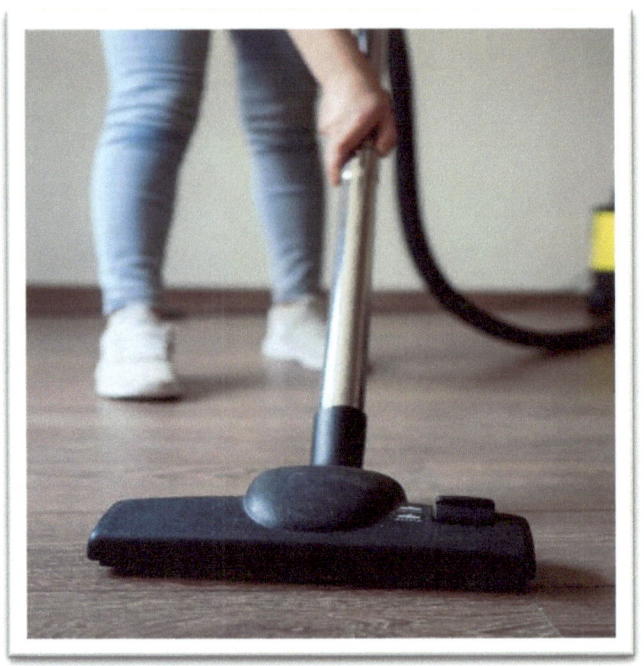

(Image by Freepik.)

A dusting powder made of diatomaceous earth and Neem also works to kill adult fleas and larvae if sprinkled over carpet and worked in with a broom, then left overnight before vacuuming again. This dusting powder may additionally be used topically on your pets before outdoor excursions; apply using a diatomaceous earth applicator (available at *Amazon* or many other online vendors), or you could also recycle a plastic ketchup bottle and use it as a natural flea powder applicator.

A SPECIES-APPROPRIATE FOOD PLAN

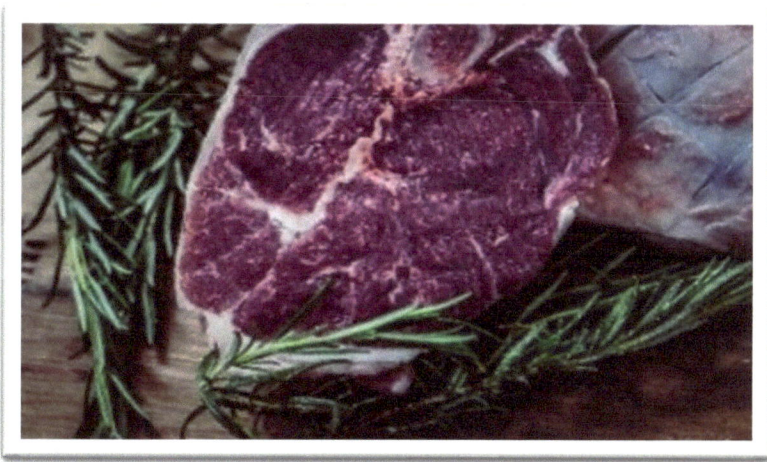

In order to thrive, animals need a diet they've genetically evolved over time to require. With pointed teeth designed to catch and shred prey for meals, dogs as well as cats are carnivores. Their digestive tracts are much shorter than plant eaters like cows, and this type of intestinal structure secretes primarily digestive enzymes that break down animal proteins and fats. From nose to tail, then, dogs and cats are designed to eat meat.

In an ideal world that honors their biological development, dogs and cats would kill and eat prey for every meal. As pets in our modern lives, dogs and cats often eat some form of dry kibble, usually in combination with canned food. Of course, not all kibble and canned food is created equallly in terms of nutritional value;

many brands are made with cheap fillers and oils (such as guar gum and canola oil) and can be high in processed ingredients, carbohydrates, and genetically modified foods.

Several fresh meat-based foods are also available commercially, which can feature ground raw bones and organ meats. Though more expensive than kibble and canned food, these raw meat-based foods can be incredibly nutritious to add to any overall dietary plan. Brands like *Viva Raw* and *We Feed Raw* make feeding a raw diet easy and convenient.

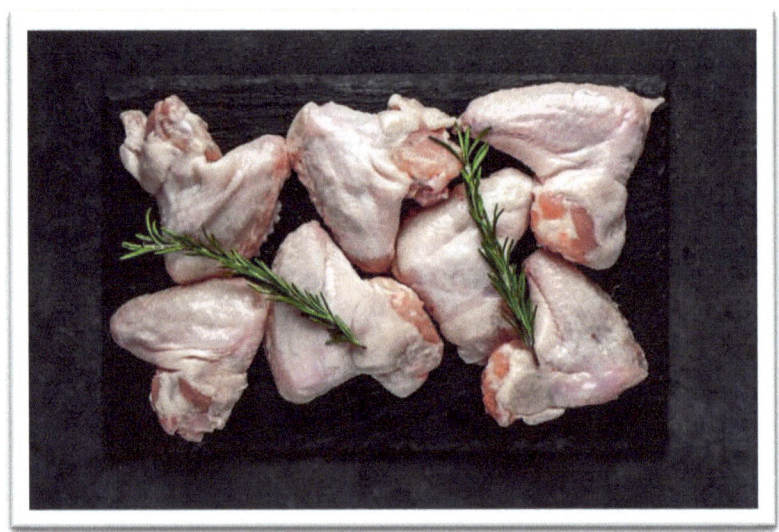

In fact, many holistically minded veterinarians who believe in species-appropriate feeding will acknowledge how choosing even as little as 20 percent of your pets' diet from raw meat-based foods will improve overall vitality.

Personally, I incorporate raw meat and/or meaty bones on a daily basis in my own dogs' nutrition plan – some days, all my dogs eat is raw meat I buy from a local farm. While ideally I believe it's best to buy organic, grass-fed beef and free-range poultry, I realize it's not always possible to source these foods. And so in my own experience, when I've not been able to find locally produced organic meats and bones, I look for whatever I can find that's as fresh and unprocessed as possible. Whenever I've lived in areas lacking farmers' markets or grocery stores selling meat and poultry sourced from local farms, I've tried to stock up and freeze as much as possible whenever I could find quality offerings.

When I was doing everything possible to boost Connell's immune system and help heal his painful skin condition, I fed him exclusively a "raw meaty bones" type of diet. (Since tripe really helped clear up his skin a number of years ago, he eats everything all my other dogs eat now – some 100% raw meat days plus some days where they eat a combination of quality kibble and canned food with bone broth and at least one raw meaty bone.) Even after so many years of following this protocol for my pups, I'm still amazed at how raw bones keep all my dogs' teeth white; also, by feeding a species-appropriate diet and keeping up with this flea and tick prevention plan, my dogs don't have "doggy breath" or any kind of "doggy body odor", either.

Another thing I've learned is how it's really important to freeze any meat (like hamburger or chicken drumsticks or turkey necks) for a minimum of three days before thawing it for dogs to eat; freezing it in this way kills bacteria and parasites to minimize microbial concerns.

While I'm sharing how I choose to feed my own animals, I always encourage any pet parents to do their own research and consult with a veterinarian about dietary options.

INGREDIENTS TO SEEK – AND ONES TO AVOID

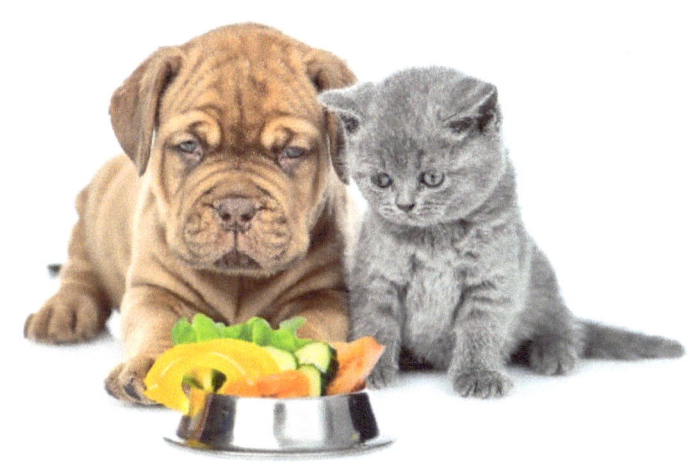

Overall, I look for kibble that's species-appropriate by being grain free and that has no genetically modified ingredients. (The online pet food retailer *Chewy* has a search option on its website that simplifies this kind of "food research".) I tend to look for kinds of kibble that are raw coated or contain raw "bits", as well as no fillers and a nice mixture of organ meats and tripe.

If you're unfamiliar with green tripe, then it's important to know it's basically raw and unprocessed animal intestines. As humans, we tend to find this concept nauseating, although most dogs love the taste! Loaded with vitamins, minerals, amino acids, essential fatty acids, probiotics, and digestive enzymes, this amazing superfood powerfully supports digestion and immunity; **truly**, as I shared earlier, it **was** green tripe that turned my golden retriever mix's health around. After about three months of adding tripe to his food, I watched his irritated skin clear – something that literally a few years and a few thousand dollars in vet visits and expensive supplements hadn't been able to address. (Many specialty grocers will carry green tripe for human consumption, but *Chewy* is once again a great place to shop if you can't find tripe locally.)

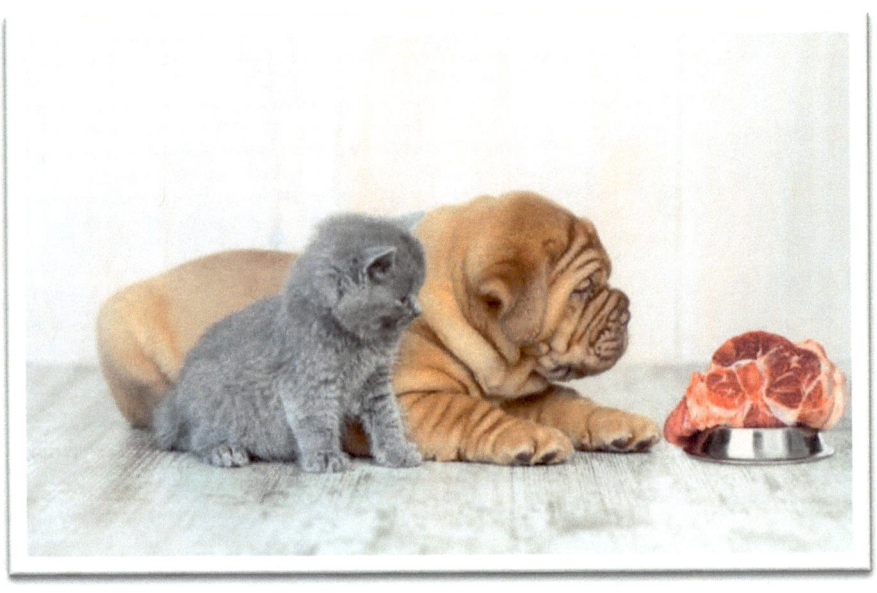

On *Chewy*, I like a few tripe brands for my fur kids very much, and I tend to rotate options (as I do with all pet foods I buy) to help prevent allergies from developing due to feeding one food too often. My dogs do particularly well with freeze-dried tripe toppers from *Ziwi Peak* and *K9 Natural*, as well as *PetKind's Bison Tripe Formula* canned food.

For foods containing raw meat and ground organs, I recommend researching locally. Yet *Chewy* does offer a wonderful variety of freeze-dried, canned, and raw-coated kibble options that can make it easy and convenient to add these species-appropriate foods into your nutrition plan. I've used so many wonderful brands from *Chewy* and *Amazon* over the years, including *Stella and Chewy's*, *Orijen*, *Open Farm*, and *The Honest Kitchen*.

SEE YOUR VETERINARIAN
IF YOU'RE UNSURE ABOUT ANYTHING

Please discontinue this protocol and be sure to seek veterinary care if you suspect any adverse reactions; remember, this information is not a substitute for sound veterinary advice. By following these suggestions, I hope you and your pets will soon be rid of unwanted fleas and ticks – easily, affordably, and naturally! (If you have any further questions or comments, you may reach me at jean@jeanbrannon.com.)

© 2024 Jean Brannon

All rights reserved. Please understand this information is shared to provide pet owners with helpful suggestions from my own experiences and in no way is meant to serve as a substitute for sound veterinary care. I recommend consulting with a compassionate, competent veterinarian before beginning this protocol. If you'd like help finding a holistically minded veterinarian in your area, please consult the following online sources:

The Academy of Veterinary Homeopathy: www.theavh.org

The American Holistic Veterinary Medical Association:

www.ahvma.org

ABOUT THE AUTHOR

Whether working with patients or the written word, licensed acupuncturist and author Jean Brannon offers ancient wisdom approaches to help people (and their pets) live their best lives. To learn more, visit her at www.jeanbrannon.com.